It's A Lifestyle...

The Link Between Tyramine
&
Migraine Headaches

It's A Lifestyle...

The Link Between Tyramine & Migraine Headaches

Mollie Newman, MS, CPT, PES, CES, Nutrition & Dietician

Owner:

Newman Coaching, LLC

Newman Coaching, LLC

2015

First Printing: 2015

ISBN 978-1-329-77782-8

Newman Coaching, LLC
9 Del Fino Place, Suite 103
Carmel Valley, CA 93924

www.newmancoaching.org

Dedication

To my world: my future husband, future baby girl, family, friends, clients, and community.

Thank you. Without your support and patience, I would have never achieved my dreams!

Dare to begin and relish in your successes!

8

How to make this a lifestyle...

Use this book as guide to living migraine free. I will give you the tools necessary to break down and rid your body of excess tyramine.

What you will gain in reading this book:
- Knowledge of what tyramine is.
- The role of Riboflavin-5-Phosphate
- Lists of High/Moderate/Low Tyramine Rich Foods
- How to keep a food journal
- How to track triggers
- Helpful delicious recipes to keep you migraine free.

It is my goal to reach out to migraine headache sufferers and offer an easy to follow guide to manage your migraine headaches. This is not a diet...this is a lifestyle!

Introduction
Personal Experience
HOW I FOUND THE SOLUTION

My first migraine headache was at the age of thirteen. It was on the second day of my first migraine headache, that my parents took me to a local doctor, who prescribed a migraine medication which was in the form of a shot called Imitrix*. This was to be injected by myself on the onset of a migraine. The major problem was catching the migraine in the 'onset', this was always the discrepancy with migraine medications that I was prescribed throughout my experience.

The excruciating pain of migraines sentenced me to three-thirteen days of living in a silent blacked-out room, relentlessly suffering from pain behind my eyes, with symptoms of vertigo, nausea, severe pain and feverish flu like symptoms. Which always sent me to the ER because it's debilitating pain.

After many cat scans, MRI's, trips to the ER and the doctor, my migraines were always ruled out to be hormonal by most professionals. I was told that I would suffer from these until my hormones changed, later in life, around the age of 25.

Not knowing any other options existed, I learned how to use the shots to 'manage' the pain, but still ended up in the ER every migraine. Where doctors would pump my body full of pain medication from Vicodin to Morphine. All of which I would later find out created headaches and migraines in the average person as they would cause withdrawal like symptoms. Along with the pain medications doctors would give me a penicillin shot, which is so rich in tyramine, it could cause a migraine on it's own. This pain staking process continued until my final migraine at the age of 21.

After many years of missing school, work and social events I was ready to explore other options and beat these migraines. My final migraine sent me to a new hospital with new doctors in Newport Beach, CA. Lucky for me, I had just moved to Newport Beach, CA to continue my college education. Finding myself blessed to have met my hero!

My hero was the Neurologist that walked into the ER that night to treat my migraine. Instead of pumping me full of pain medication on first sight; he asked questions: How long I've been in pain? Have I been nauseated? Have you had a migraine before? What do you take for your migraines? And the questions streamed a long. In excruciating pain I almost preferred the pain medication rather than have to talk to this doctor.

It wasn't until he began to explain that he may have a solution for me, through a more holistic approach to treat my migraines.

The light bulb went off for me when he asked, "Have you ever heard of food related migraines?" This was something that seemed to make perfect sense, but I had never heard about diet being a possible cause of my migraines. He proceeded to tell me with a smile that they were performing an experimental study through a local California State College on food related migraines. He thought I was a perfect candidate with being young, having the strong history of migraine headaches and open to any possible treatment.

Through this experimental study they would take out all tyramine from participants' diet and slowly introduce the tyramine foods back into their diet as if they were an infant learning to eat solids. One food at a time over an extended range of days to be sure there was no negative reaction.

The neurologist then proceeded to explain that he would send me home with a list of tyramine free foods of which I was to follow for one week. To my surprise my neurologist did not pump me full of medication rather he hooked me up to an IV to rehydrate my body. Sent me home with this 'magic' list and said call my office to arrange a follow-up appointment in one week. Once you get home you should be able to take Advil* as needed for the pain. I was stunned that A)I got sent home still in tremendous pain and B) that there could possibly be a life without migraine headaches. I was skeptical, but his eyes and theory were so reassuring that I trusted this may be my miracle answer.

Upon my release from the hospital still in immense pain and prescribed to rest, take Advil* as needed for pain and only eat food on this list that my neurologist had typed himself titled *Tyramine Free Food*. I took this time to trust in his theory and ride out this migraine as prescribed. Two days later I was on my journaling track, migraine free and thus far tyramine free.

Anyone who has suffered from a migraine knows that its like chasing a unicorn to find a solution or cure for migraine headaches. You want to find an answer to the cause of your migraine and be able to treat them before they get too severe. I thought, "Why not? I have tried literally everything else. If I can control my migraines through diet, it would be miraculous! I was ready to do whatever it took!

The purpose of this book is to share my experience because everyone deserves to know about tyramine and the relief that this lifestyle can bring.

I want to encourage you to live migraine free with a focus on all the things you can have in your diet rather than the overwhelming list of the things you cannot have. As I believe it is important to live a rich life all in moderation!

Chapter 1
How I got rid of migraines:
Step by step

The migraine study that I took part in was one of my most life changing experiences. We began with a questionnaire about migraines with simple questions about my triggers, treatments and family history of migraines.

After answering the standard group of questions, I was sent home with homework of keeping a one week food journal. My journal was honest and tracked every item that entered my body.

The doctors found it interesting that although I ate a healthy diet of fresh, unprocessed foods, I was eating some foods that are major triggers and were very high in tyramine. We evaluated all of the foods and drinks from the week, which is the course of action I recommend for you, as explained in Chapter 7.

When you have completed your first week of eating only foods on the list from Chapter 6. You must begin journaling week two by adding one to three items per week, from the lists in Chapters 4-5. Be sure to log your reactions to these introduced foods and track if they are triggers or safe to eat.

Everyone has different body chemistry so keep in mind what works for you may not work for someone else. This is what makes this process so unique.

On week two you can introduce the enzyme Riboflavin-5-Phosphate into your daily diet. Chapter 3 will discuss the benefits of Riboflavin-5-Phosphate.

During this process that begins in week two, you must track everything that you put in your mouth, even the water you consume throughout the day. You are not focusing on your diet for weight loss in this effort. You are tracking for migraine triggers, so be honest and thorough in recording everything you eat and drink. Note the food, and the 'condition' it is in. If you are eating fruits and vegetables, note if they are under-ripe, over-ripe, canned, froze, etc.

Choose your favorite food and introduce them to your diet first. For this, I chose avocado first, and to my surprise, the solid green meat of the avocados gave me no residual problems. However, the avocados that were overripe (with brown spots throughout) effected my headaches. Introduce food slowly, so you can see if they have an affect on you. This is highly important in this journey. The slow introduction of tyramine foods will take time, but you will see benefits as you will learn your triggers. Eventually in time even without journaling, you will become very in-tuned with your body. You will recognize that when you feel sluggish with a faint headache, you may be suffering from a slow build up of tyramine and need to lighten up on the tyramine rich foods.

In my experience being diligent about taking the R5P, two (2/d) a day, my body and mind felt clear and I began to eat tyramine rich foods with no residual effects. This is what you eventually want, to live migraine free and able to enjoy the foods you love.

If you follow this regimen, you will find what works best with your body, along with living a healthier cleaner lifestyle.

You are most likely going to find that you will be shopping around the perimeter of the grocery store, and leaving those high sodium and preserved foods in the middle of the store for others to purchase. My best advise for migraines sufferers to understand that this is a process and can take great patience. For some, the results will be seen in an instant. For others, it will take time to rid your body of the built up tyramine.

If you follow the prescribed path you will find yourself with more energy and living migraine free, as I have for the past 12 years.

Chapter 2
What is Tyramine?

Tyramine is an amino acid that is created during the breakdown of a protein. That breakdown occurs as food is ripened, dried, fermented, cured, pickled, canned or preserved.

Tyramine is naturally produced in the human gallbladder. In migraine sufferers, there is a build up of tyramine that the body cannot break down on it's own. Migraine sufferers are deficient in the enzyme Riboflavin-5-Phosphate. With this deficiency, the body goes into attack mode and blood pressure rises, causing swelling of the blood vessels that surround the cranial cavity, causing the beginnings of the feared migraine.

When there is too much tyramine in the system, it is important to keep sodium intake down, as the body will react with a stronger migraine since your blood pressure will be elevated from high levels of sodium. A good guideline is to keep within the recommended daily intake of 2,300 mg of sodium a day.

Stress produces a similar trigger to this reaction as blood pressure rises with increased stress. Migraines can be worsened with outside stressors, such as work, relationships, school and general day-to-day life challenges. Stress is one of the leading killers in the United States and is often cited as a contributing factor to many fatal diseases.

Another factor increasing the chances of migraine is too much screen time. The white back light is damaging to the retina and leads to focusing without blinking for long periods of time.

Migraine sufferers need to limit exposure to high levels of tyramine, stress and screen time! Adding a supplement of Riboflavine-5-Phosphate (R5P) to your daily routine will help you achieve a migraine free life.

Keep in mind, exercise is great for overall health and helps promote healthy digestion by aiding in breaking down tyramine levels. Take 30 minutes a day to do something active and get your blood flowing.

Chapter 3
Riboflavin-5-Phosphate

In working with many professionals throughout my migraine history, it was not until I went to my chiropractor, Wilson E Smith DC PhD, who introduced the concept of supplementing Riboflavin-5-Phosphate (R5P) into my daily diet.

At this point in my life I was eating a very low tyramine diet at the age of 28 and happy to report I was migraine free. Wilson Smith suggested that I could take R5P and re introduce without fear some of the tyramine rich food I had been avoiding for years.

He further explained that R5P helps aid in the break down of tyramine. Our body naturally produces tyramine in the gallbladder. In migraines sufferers the R5P helps keep tyramine at a tolerable level.

Interested to see if his suggestion would work, I followed the recommendation of supplementing R5P and took 2 (2/d) dietary supplements daily and began introducing more tyramine rich foods to my diet. To my surprise, taking R5P allowed me to eat everything from the lists in Chapter 5-6 and introduce majority of the foods listed in Chapter 4. Finding this combination of diet and supplementation was the turning point for me living migraine free.

With supplementing R5P into the daily diet one would be able to eat moderate amounts of tyramine. Introduce tyramine foods slowly into diet as it will be a test to see what your body reacts to. Each person's body chemistry is different which makes introducing foods slowly a key factor in this process. Be cautious as the introduction will not be an instant migraine, but it is due to a build of tyramine in the body that will cause a migraine.

Foods high in R5P that should be added into your diet are: beets greens, almonds, soybeans, spinach, yogurt, mushrooms, eggs, asparagus and lean meats, such as fish, white chicken meat, white turkey meat, etc.

In the next chapters foods with tyramine will be introduced to help you with your journey to living migraine free.

Chapter 4
Foods to Avoid

The following list will be completely overwhelming as it may include many of your favorite foods, the key thing to remember is you are following this to avoid suffering from another migraine. This is incentive enough to give up many things!

Aged Cheeses: (Avoid all aged cheeses, Blue, Smoked Cheese, or Hard Cheese)	Cheddar, Blue, Gorgonzola, Camembert, Brie, Stilton, Swiss, Feta, Colby, Boursalt, Gouda, Gruyere, Roquefort, Provolone, Emmentaler, Parmesan, Muenster, Romano, All non pasteurized cheese
Dairy & Egg	Quiche, Protein dietary supplements w/ yeast extract
Aged, fermented, smoked, air dried, cured, processed and pickled meats: Luncheon meats containing nitrites and nitrates	Mortadella, Pepperoni, Salami, Summer Sausage, Jerky, Pancetta, Prosciutto, Bacon, Liverwurst, Liver, Sausage, Bologna, Cured Ham, Hot Dogs, Corned Beef, Poultry Skin, Game Meats
Fish	Lox, Anchovies, Roe, Herring, Caviar, Sardines, Cafelta Fish, Shrimp Paste, Fish Sauce

Fruits: Fermented, Canned, Dried, Overripeness	Avocado(Browned), Banana (Browned), Date, Dragon Fruit, Fig, Raisin, Cranberry, Guava, Lychee, Mango Passion Fruit, Papaya, Persimmon, Currents, Preserves
Vegetables: Fermented, Canned, Dried, Overripeness	Ancho Chili, Beet, Broad Bean, Fava Bean, Raw Garlic, Olives, Turnip, Bean Sprout, Navy Beans, Raw Onions, Daikon, Ginger, Parsnip, Rutabaga, Sauerkraut, Jicama, Jerusalem Artichoke, Taro, Water Chestnut
Breads: Fermented yeast, Brewers Yeast, Yeats Extract	Sourdough, Soda Bread, Coffee Cake, Raisin Bread, Banana Bread
Fats, Oils, and Misc.	Vinegars: Balsamic, White Wine, Red Wine, Apple Cider Tahini, Marmite, Vegemite, Liquid Smoke,Fermented Soy: Tofu, Soy Sauce, Soy Paste, Miso, Teriyaki Sauce,Ingredients on Food Labels: Monosodium Glutamate (MSG), Nitrates, Nitrites, Sulfites, Aspartame, Sulfur, High Fructose Corn Syrup
Alcohol Wine (Longer the juice has contact with the skin, the more tyramine)Listed to the right Highest tyramine to lowest	All beers bottled or canned including non alcoholic beers, Ciders...Red Wines: Zinfandel. Cabernet Sauvignon, Cab Franc, Merlot, Malbec,Pinot Noir, Rose White Wines: Chardonnay, Sauvignon Blanc, Chenin Blanc, Pinot Grigio, Verdejo, Champagne Hard Alcohols: (Anything that says aged or anejo) Rum, Tequila, Scotch, Whiskey, Bourbon, Sheri, Marsala, Any and all mixers that are not "fresh squeezed".
Cocoa	Brownies, Chocolate Cake, Lava Cake, Chocolate Ice Cream/Milkshake, Mole Sauce, Dark/Milk Chocolate, Hot Chocolate, Pudding, Mouse

Chapter 5
Foods to Consume in Moderation

These food should be consumed in moderation and slowly introduced first into your diet. This means you should get away with having servings of the following foods every other day without too much tyramine build up.

Cheese	Ailsa Craig, Babybel, Ricotta, Cotija, Galbani, Paneer, Breakfast cheese, Mozzarella, Goat Cheese, Marscapone, Monet, Queso Fresco
Dairy & Egg	Egg Nog, Flan, Brule, Rice pudding, Tapioca
Meats	Beef, Turkey, Nitrate/Nitrite Free Uncured Bacon/Ham/Sausage, Lamb, Duck, Venison, Elk, Bison
Fish	Carp, Catfish, Cobia, Cod, Conch, Croaker, Dolphinfish, Drum, Grouper, Herring, Lingcod, Mackerel, Marlin, Menhaden, Milkfish, Monkfish, Mullet, Opah, Orange Roughy, Octopus, Paddlefish, Perch, Pike, Pollock, Sablefish, Scallop, Shark, Smelt, Spearfish, Sturgeon, Swordfish, Tilefish, Toothfish, Tuna, Wahoo, Walleye, Whitefish, Wreckfish,

Foods to Consume in Moderation Continued...

Fruits	Jam, Jelly, Kiwi,
Vegetables	Brussel Sprouts, Acorn Squash, Butternut Squash, Spaghetti Squash, Pumpkin
Breads	Cereals with dried fruit, Morning Glory Bread, Pound Cake,
Fats, Oils, and Misc.	
Alcohol	Champagne and Vodka

Chapter 6
Foods to Consume Freely

These food contain little or no tyramine which make them easier to digest. These should be consumed fresh meaning you are eating these foods, as close to their natural state as possible.

Cheese	American Cheese, Cottage Cheese, Cream Cheese, Fresh Mozzarella, Fromage, Farm Chevre, Fresh Ricotta, Primo Fresca, Velveeta
Dairy & Egg	Eggs, Milk: Cream, Whole, 2%, 1% or Skim, Butter, Ice Cream, Yogurt, Sour Cream,
Meats	Chicken, Grass Fed Beef, Pork
Fish	Abalone, Alfonsino, Anchovy, Bass, Butterfish, Clams, Crab, Crawfish, Dab, Eel, Flounder, Halibut, Krill, Lobster, Mussels, Oysters, Pomfret, Pompano, Salmon, Sanddao, Sardine, Sea bass, Sea Urchin, Sea trout, Seaweed, Shrimp, Snapper, Sole, Squid, Tilapia, Trout,

Foods to Consume Freely Continued...

Fruit

Acia, Aceola, Apple, Apricots, Avocado (Green), Banana (Green), Blackberry, Blueberries, Camu Camu Berry, Cherries, Coconut, Cucumber, Goji Berries, Gooseberry, Grapefruit, Grapes, Jackfruit, Kumquat, Lemon, Lime, Lucuma, Mangosteen, Melon, Nectarine, Orange, Peach, Pear, Pineapple, Plum, Pomegranate, Prickly Pear, Strawberries, Tangerine/ Clementine, Watermelon

Vegetables

Artichoke, Arugula, Asparagus, Eggplant, Amaranth, Legumes: Alfalfa Sprout, Azuki Beans, Black Beans, Black-Eye peas, Chickpeas, Green Beans, Kidney Beans, Lentils, Mung Beans, Pinto Beans, Navy Beans, Runner Beans, Split Peas, Soy Beans, Peas, Snap Peas (Not to Pod just the pea), Bock Choy, Broccoflower, Broccoli, Cabbage, Calabrese, Cannabis, Carrots, Cauliflower, Celery, Chard, Collard Greens, Corn Salad, Endive, Fiddleheads, Frisee, Herbs/Spices: Anise, Basil, Caraway, Cilantro, Chamomile, Dill, Fennel, Lavender, Lemon Grass, Marjoram, Oregano, Parsley, Rosemary, Sage, Thyme, Kale, Kohlrabi, Lettuce, Corn, Mushrooms, Mustard Greens, Nettles, New Zealand Spinach, Okra, Chives, Green Onion, Parsley, Peppers: Bell Pepper, Chili Pepper, Jalepano, Habanero, Paprika, Tabasco Pepper, Cayenne Pepper, Radicchio, Rhubarb, Beet Greens, Radish, Wasabi, White Radish, Zucchini, Banana Squash, Gem Squash, Marrow Squash, Patty Pans, Tat Soi, Tomato, Sweet Potato, Potato, Yam, Watercress

Chapter 7
First Week Journal

Now that we have reviewed through the lists of foods from which you should avoid, eat in moderation and eat freely, here is your opportunity to start fighting your migraines. If you choose to take the R5P then you would begin now. Below is an example of how your journal should look: Be sure to log even your water intake!

First Week Food Journal Entry	
Date	
Day of the week	
Weather:	
Mood:	
How does your body feel?	
Breakfast:	
Snack:	

Lunch:	
Snack:	
Dinner:	
Snack:	

Chapter 8
Tyramine Journal Week 2 and On

This journal will read very similar to the first week, with the additional instruction to include all ingredients. It will seem like it takes more time, but believe me it will be worth it once your migraines are gone! Here is a sample layout and I will include a sample of my personal journal to help as a guide:

Tyramine Journal Entry	
Date	
Day of the week	
Weather:	
Mood:	
Tyramine Introduced:	
How does your body feel?	
Breakfast:	

Snack:	
Lunch:	
Snack:	
Dinner:	
Snack:	

Here is the sample of one of my journal entries when I began to log for the tyramine study:

Sample: Tyramine Journal Entry	
Date:	September 14, 2002
Day of Week:	Saturday
Weather:	Sunny Surf Day, Plenty of Vitamin D!
Mood:	Feeling Great
Tyramine Introduced:	Introduced: Balsamic Vinegar & Raw Onion (not my friends)
How does your body feel?	I feel really good today it's been 3 weeks since I began.
Breakfast:	2 Egg whites, 1/4 avocado & 1/2 cup chopped tomato. Water and Orange Juice
Snack:	No snack, just water

Lunch:	Sandwich: BBQ Chicken, homemade BBQ sauce(ketchup, brown sugar, mccormick steak seasoning, brown sugar, and rosemary) lettuce, tomato, raw onion (pulled of instant reaction- not normal), mayonnaise, mustard. Water
Snack:	Water and cocktail (vodka, soda water, splash of fresh mango puree)
Dinner:	Baked Potato with butter, sour cream, chives and salt and pepper, Grilled Chicken w/lemon butter and caramelized onion (cook onion is ok), Salad, Iceberg, apple, carrot, avocado with homemade salad dressing (olive oil, maple syrup, salt, pepper, garlic, thyme, oregano).
Snack:	Water and cocktail (vodka, soda water, fresh slice lime)

It was helpful for the study and for me to include the way I was feeling. If I had a reaction, I put it in the journal. This way you get a very clear picture and if you feel any reactions from the food you have eaten it the next day include this in your journal as well.

Chapter 9
Low Tyramine Breakfast Recipes

Here are a few low tyramine recipes that I have created over the past twelve years. Cooking has always been a passion of mine, I hope you find these recipes helpful.

Pancakes

Ingredients...

1 1/2 Cups	All-Purpose Flour
3 1/2 Tbsp	Baking Powder
2 Tbsp	White Sugar
1 1/4 Cup	Whole Milk
1 Whole	Egg
3 Tbsp	Salted Butter

Directions: Combine all dry ingredients in sifter and sift into a large mixing bowl. Slowly add milk, egg and melted butter and mice until smooth. If too thick add milk 1Tbsp at a time. Pour onto griddle over medium heat. Brown both sides and serve with butter, fresh strawberries and powdered sugar.

Oatmeal

Ingredients...

1 Cup	Cooked Organic Oatmeal
1/2 Cup	Chopped Apple
1 Tsp	Cinnamon
1 Tbsp	Local Honey
1/4 Cups	Chopped Walnuts (Can be reactive tyramine medium in walnuts)

Directions: Over cooked oatmeal, add toppings of apple, cinnamon, honey and walnuts, enjoy hot!

Classic Smoothy

Ingredients...

1 Cup	Organic Whole Milk Plain Yogurt
1 Scoop	Organic Brown Rice Protein Powder
1 Medium	Green/Bright Yellow Banana
1/2 Cup	Frozen Strawberry (I buy them fresh and freeze them/The max they are in the freezer is one week)
1 Cup	Fresh Squeezed Orange Juice

Directions: Put all ingredients in a blender and spend until smooth.

Good Morning Toast

Ingredients...

1/2 Whole	Green Avocado (no brown spots they should be slightly hard/without brown spots or soft spots)
1 Whole	Farm Fresh Egg
1 Slice	Ezekiel Whole Wheat Bread
1 Tsp	Salted butter

Direction: Toast bread and butter, slice avocado over buttered toast and add egg cooked over easy and dash with salt and pepper.

Eggs-n-Toast

Ingredients...

2 Large	Farm Fresh Eggs
2 Slices	Ezekiel Whole Wheat Bread
1 Tbsp	Butter
Dash	Salt and Pepper

Directions: Toast bread, over low heat crack eggs in lightly greased pan (I use olive oil), flip once egg whites no longer runny and flip cook for 30 seconds for runny yolks. Butter toast and cut into small squares, place eggs over and serve.

Omelette

Ingredients...

3 Large	Farm Fresh Eggs
1/4 Cup	Onion
1/4 Cup	Zucchini
1/4 Cup	Mushroom

Directions: Scramble eggs set aside, sauté onion, zucchini, mushrooms in olive oil until onion is clear over medium heat, lower heat to low and pour eggs over sautéed veggies and flip...add fresh cheese if preferred and serve.

Parfait

Ingredients...

2 Cups	Organic Whole Milk Plain Yogurt
1/2 Cup	Fresh cut Strawberries
1/2 Cup	Fresh Blueberries
1/2 Cup	Green/Bright Yellow Banana Chopped
1 Tbsp	Local Fresh Honey

Directions: In bowl pour half of the yogurt layer fruit. Pour remaining yogurt over fruit and drizzle with honey.

Chapter 10
Low Tyramine Lunch Recipes

Turkey Meat Cups	
Ingredients...	
1 Pound	Turkey Meat
1/2 Whole	Red onion chopped
6 Whole	Mushrooms chopped
Drizzle	Olive oil
1 Whole	Egg
1 Tbsp	McCormick Steak Seasoning

Directions: Preheat oven to 375 degrees. In sauté pan add olive oil, red onion and mushrooms. Cook until onions are clear. Put to side off heat. In medium mixing bowl combine Turkey meat, cooked onion and mushrooms, raw egg and seasoning. Combine with wooden spoon or get your hands dirty and press together until thoroughly combined.

Divide into un-greased muffin tin, filling each round 3/4 of the way. Place in oven and bake for 10 minutes, should be browned all of the way through, if still pink place back in oven and bake an additional 5 minutes. Let cool and keep in fridge for easy high protein snack or lunch.

Lettuce Wraps

Ingredients...

4 Slices	Nitrate/Nitrate/Sulfite/Uncured Turkey meat
4 Lettuce Leaf	Iceberg or Red Leaf
4 Slices	Fresh Mozzarella Cheese
4 Slices	Tomato
2 Tbsp	Dijon Mustard

Directions: On each lettuce leaf, layer mustard, turkey, cheese and tomato. Roll and serve.

Chicken Salad

Ingredients...

2 Cup	Cubed-Grilled Chicken Breast
1/4 Cup	Celery
1/2 Cup	Cut in Half -Red Grapes
4 Tbspn	Mayonaise
Dash	Salt and Pepper

Directions: Combine: Grill chicken - let cool then cut into cubes, chop celery, grapes, and mayonnaise in medium mixing bowl. Add Salt and Pepper to Taste. Serve on whole wheat crackers, as a sandwich, or in lettuce wraps.

Cottage Cheese Bowl

Ingredients...

1 Cup	Cubed Grilled Chicken
2 Cups	Organic Whole Milk Cottage Cheese
1/2 Whole	Sliced Tomato
1/2 Whole	Avocado (Green) Diced
Dash	Salt and pepper

Directions: In a Bowl layer cottage cheese, tomato, avocado, chicken and dash with salt and pepper to taste.

Taco Salad

Ingredients...

1 Cup	Chopped Lettuce
1/2 Cup	Cooked Ground Turkey
Drizzle	Olive oil
Dash	Salt and Pepper
1/2 Cup	Cut Corn off the cob
1/2 Whole	Avocado (Green)
3 Tbsp	Organic Whole Milk Sour Cream
3 Tbsp	Salsa (Ch.13)
3 Sprigs	Cilantro chopped

Directions: Cook Turkey meat in sauté can drizzled with olive oil, dash with salt and pepper for taste (If you like spice add in red pepper chili flakes-1 Tsp). Cook until solid in color. In a bowl combine all ingredients layering from top to bottom then toss with sour cream and salsa. Garnish with Cilantro

Cobb Salad

Ingredients...

1 Cup	Chopped Lettuce
1/2 Cup	Shredded Purple Cabbage
1/4 Cup	Shredded Carrots
1/2 Whole	Apple chopped
1/2 Whole	Tomato Chopped
1 Whole	Hard Boiled Egg - Chopped
2 Slices	Uncured/Nitrate/Nitrate/Unsmoked bacon-cooked and chopped
2-3 Tbsp	Homemade Italian Dressing (Ch.13)

Directions: In a bowl combine all ingredients layering from top to bottom then toss with salad dressing.

Open-Face Bagel

Ingredients...

1 Whole	Poppyseed Bagel (Fresh from bakery)
2 Tbsp	Organic Whole Cream Cheese Plain
1 Half	Sliced Tomato
Dash	Italian Dried Herbs or Fresh Basil (4 leaves chopped)
Dash	Salt and pepper

Directions: Toast bagel cut in half, spread cream cheese, layer tomatoes and garnish with herbs, salt and pepper.

Chapter 11
Low Tyramine Dinner Recipes

Salmon Skewers

Ingredients...

1 Pound	Fresh Wild Salmon Cubed
1 Bunch	Basil Chopped
2 Tbsp	Salted Butter
Dash	Salt and Pepper
2 Cups	Fresh Corn of the cob cut
1/4 Cup	Diced Mushrooms
1/4 Cup	Shopped Red onion
2 Tbsp	Olive Oil

Directions: Place cubed salmon onto skewers, lightly salt and pepper. Grill for 3 minutes each side. Let stand off heat while you prep the rest.

Sauté in medium pan over medium heat, olive oil, half the basil, mushrooms and onion. Cook until Onions are clear. In small sauté pan add butter, basil and salt & pepper, let simmer until butter is almost browned.

Place skewers on plate drizzle butter mixture over the salmon skewers, serve over bed of corm mixture. Enjoy!

Fish Tacos

Ingredients...

1.5 Pounds	White Fish (Halibut, Talapia, Trout, etc)
2 Tbsp	MSG/Sodium Free Cajun Spice
2 Tbsp	Olive oil
8 Leaf	Red Cabbage (they will form cups)
1 Whole	Avocado (Green) thinly sliced
8 Tbsp	Organic Whole Milk Sour Cream

Directions: In large saute pan heat olive oil over medium heat, add fish and cajun spices, break apart fish as it cooks so it is shredded rather than whole fish. Cook until solid white all of the way through.

Place 4 cabbage cups on each plate, fill equally with cooked cajun fish, layer sliced avocado, and fish off with sour cream. Enjoy!

Halibut over Bed of Spinach

Ingredients...

6 oz (per serving)	Fresh Caught Halibut
Drizzle	Olive Oil
1 Whole	Shallot chopped
1 Tsp	Red Pepper Chili Flakes
1 Bunch	Fresh Basil (Chopped)
1 Whole	Meyer Lemon
1 Clove	Minced Garlic

Directions:In saute pan drizzle with olive oil, add shallot, red pepper chili flakes, and basil sauté oil shallots are clear. Add to sauté pan halibut cook 4-5 minutes on both sides, squeeze 1/2 meyer lemon into pan.

In another pan sauté spinach with half meyer lemon, garlic, olive oil until wilted. Place bed of spinach onto plate, pour halibut with stock over and serve.

Shrimp Pasta

Ingredients...

1 Dozen	Prawns
1 Whole	Zucchini Chopped
1 Whole	Red Onion Chopped
1 Bunch	Fresh Basil (chopped)
1 Tbsp	Red Pepper Chilli Flakes
1/4 Cup	Olive Oil
3 Cups	Fresh Linguini

Directions: In stock pot boil 6 cups water. In large sauté pan combine: Zucchini, Onion, Basil (leave some out for garnish), Chili flakes, olive oil, salt and pepper. Sauté until the onions are clear and add prawns.

Add Fresh linguini into boiling stock pot of water and cook 7-10 minutes until tender.

Sauté prawns and veggies until both sides of prawns are solid white for about 2 minutes each side over medium heat. Add cooked pasta and marry together. Then serve and garnish with extra fresh basil.

Roasted Chicken

Ingredients...

1 Whole	No hormone added Chicken
1 Whole	Red onion
1 Whole	Orange
3 Sprigs	Fresh Rosemary
Dash	Salt and Pepper
2 Whole	Yukon Gold potatoes - chopped
3 Cups	String Beans (Fresh Green Beans
Drizzle	Olive Oil
Dash	Salt and pepper

Directions: Preheat oven 375 degrees. Rinse under cold fresh water the whole chicken. Stuff with red onion, Orange and 2 sprigs of rosemary. Salt and Pepper entire top of chicken. Roast in oven for 1 hour 30minutes. In separate pan add potatoes, chop one sprig of rosemary toss in olive oil and dash salt and pepper. Roast for 45-60 minutes in same oven.
   In sauté pan add string beans, drizzle with olive oil and add salt and pepper for flavor. Over medium heat sauté staring occasionally for even heat throughout, cook until tender.

Chapter 12
Low Tyramine Snack Recipes

Hummus Dip	
Ingredients...	
3 Cups	Cooked Garbanzo Beans
1 Clove	Minced Garlic
1/4 Cup	Olive Oil
Dash	Salt and Pepper

Directions: Combine all ingredients into blender or food processor and pulse until the hummus is smooth in texture.

For more flavors try adding: Avocado (Green), Basil, Roasted Garlic or Bell Peppers (only if you don't get a reaction).

Serve with: Fresh Cut veggies and enjoy a high protein healthy snack.

Edamame

Ingredients...

1 Pound	Boiled Soy Beans in Pod
1 Tbsp	Salted Butter
1 Clove	Garlic
Dash	Salt and Pepper

Directions:Boils soy beans in pod, Strain from water add to large sauté pan. Combine butter, garlic, soy beans and lightly salt and pepper. Sauté over medium heat for 5-7 minutes stirring occasionally, so all pods are coated. Then serve warm.

Apple with Peanut Butter

Ingredients...

2 Cups	Raw Peanuts
2 Tbsp	Local Honey
1 Whole	Apple
Dash	Cinnamon

Directions: Combine Peanuts and honey in blender or food processor to make the peanut butter, add more honey to taste. Slice apples and smear peanut butter over each slice, dash with cinnamon and serve.

Trail Mix

Ingredients...

1 Cup	Raw Almonds
1 Cup	Raw Walnuts
1 Cup	Raw Pecans
1 Cup	White Chocolate Chips
1 Cup	Dried Apricot (If you do not have a reaction) Dice and add to mix.

Directions:In a large bowl combine all ingredients and separate into small snack backs for an easy and healthy snack on the go!

Chapter 13
Low Tyramine Dressing, Sauce & Marinade Recipes

Salsa	
Ingredients...	
3 Cups	Chopped Tomatoes
1/2 Cup	Chopped Red Onion (Saute until clear)
2 Clove	Minced Garlic
1 Bundle	Fresh Cilantro Chopped
2 Tbsp	McCormick* Steak Seasoning

Directions: Place all in blender or food processor and pulse until combined, for chunky salsa pulse a few times and for liquid salsa, pulse until fluid.

BBQ Sauce

Ingredients...

2 Cups	Organic No Sodium Ketchup
1/2 Cup	Light Brown Sugar
2 Sprigs	Fresh minced Rosemary
2 Tbsp	McCormick* Steak Seasoning
2 Cloves	Minced Garlic

Directions: Add all ingredient into medium sauce pan and whisk together until begins to boil. Remove from heat and store in refrigerator for up to 2 weeks. Use over your favorite grilled meats!

Italian Salad Dressing

Ingredients...

1 Cup	Olive oil
1 Clove	Minced Garlic
2 Tbsp	Fresh Chopped Oregano
2 Tbsp	Fresh Chopped English Thyme
1/2 Whole	Squeezed Meyer Lemon
2 Tbsp	Local Honey
To taste	Salt and Pepper

Directions: Combine all ingredients in blender or food processor and pulse until all ingredients blend. Keep on refrigerator up to 2 weeks.

Apricot & Peach Marinade

Ingredients...

1/2 Cup	Minced Fresh Apricot
1/2 Cup	Minced Fresh Peach
2 Tbsp	Salted Butter
Dash	Salt and Pepper

Directions: Combine in small sauté pan over low heat until fruit is soft and completely broken down. Pour over your favorite pork, chicken, fish or wild game dish!

Chapter 14
Hidden Names to Watch For in the Grocery Store

Artificial Flavors
Enriched Wheat
Hydrogenated or Fractioned oils
Monosodium Glutamate (MSG)
High Fructose Corn Syrup
Potassium Benzoate and Sodium Sodium Benzoate
Artificial Coloring
Acesulfame-K
Sucralose
Aspartame
BHA and BHT
Propyl Gallate
Soy
Soy Lecithin
Potassium Sorbate
Polysorbate 80
Canola Oil

Chapter 15
Journaling Space For You

My Triggers Are...

My Triggers Are...

Headache Log....

Date/Time/Trigger/Length/Severity/Treatment

Headache Log....

Date/Time/Trigger/Length/Severity/Treatment

Recipes you created...

Recipes you created...

Recipes you created...

Notes...

Notes...

Notes...

www.ingramcontent.com/pod-product-compliance
Lightning Source LLC
Chambersburg PA
CBHW020408290526
45785CB00005B/2471